I0843786

Table of Contents

PREVIEW

GERD, diarrhea and colorectal cancer are examples of gastrointestinal diseases. When examined, some diseases show nothing wrong with the GI tract, but there are still symptoms. Other diseases have symptoms, and there are also visible irregularities in the GI tract. Most gastrointestinal diseases can be prevented and/or treated.

Gastrointestinal diseases affect the gastrointestinal (GI) tract from the mouth to the anus. There are two types: functional and structural. Some examples include nausea/vomiting, food poisoning, lactose intolerance and diarrhea.

BREAKFAST

1. Breakfast Casserole with Cheese Sauce

Prep Time: 25 Minutes

Cook Time: 30 Minutes

Servings: 24

Ingredients

- two 11x8 or 9x13 baking pans

Scrambled Eggs:

- 18 eggs
- 1 cup milk
- 1/2 tsp salt and pepper
- Casserole Toppings:
- 4 Tbsp oil (for greasing pans)
- 30 oz hash browns
- 1 lb breakfast sausage (browned and crumbled in a skillet)
- 3 slices ham (chopped)

- 1/4 cup bacon (crumbled bacon bits)
- Cheese Sauce:
- 4 Tbsp unsalted butter
- 1/4 cup flour
- 2 cups milk
- 3/4 tsp salt
- 1 tsp sugar
- 3/4 tsp white pepper
- 1/2 tsp dry mustard
- 2 cups cheddar cheese (grated)

Instructions

1. Preheat the oven to 350°F. Grease two pans with 2 tbsp of oil each. Set aside.

2. Whisk the eggs, milk, salt, and pepper in a large bowl. Heat a large skillet or griddle over medium heat and grease with the fat from the cooked sausage. Pour your egg mixture into the skillet and scramble until set. Set aside.

3. To Make Cheese Sauce: In a small saucepan melt butter and whisk in the flour. Add milk and bring to a simmer. Stir in the remaining ingredients and heat until thickened.

4. Evenly arrange Casseroles in the following order: hashbrowns, sausage, bacon, eggs, and cheese sauce. Arrange the second casserole in the same order using ham.

5. how to make ahead a breakfast casserole

6. Bake for 25-40 minutes or until steaming hot. Freeze or keep the second casserole for a make-ahead breakfast.

Prep Time: 10 Minutes

Cook Time: 10 Minutes

Servings: 16

Ingredients

Equipment:

- two cast-iron skillets (9 or 10.5-inches)
- mixing bowl
- measuring cup
- pizza cutter or dough scraper

Quick Pizza Dough:

- 1 1/4 cup warm water
- 1 Tbsp heaping yeast
- 1 Tbsp heaping sugar
- 2 tsp salt
- 4 Tbsp oil
- 3 3/4 cups flour

Pizza Toppings:

- 2 cups sausage gravy

- 3 cups Monterey Jack Colby cheese (or half mozzarella and cheddar cheese)
- 9 scrambled eggs
- pinch of ground sage (optional)

Instructions

1. Make the pizza crust: in a pint measuring cup, whisk together the yeast, sugar, warm water, salt, and oil. Let sit 5 minutes to foam. Pour into the flour and form dough into a ball. The dough is ready when it no longer sticks to your hands.
2. Divide the dough into two well-greased cast-iron pans: spread about 1 cup of sausage gravy over each crust. Top each pizza with 1 1/2 cups cheese and scrambled eggs. Sprinkle the top with a pinch of ground sage.
3. Bake: in a pre-heated 500°F for 7-10 minutes or until crust is browned and the pizza is done.

Prep Time: 15 Minutes

Cook Time: 40 Minutes

Servings: 8

Ingredients

- 9-inch pie pan
- 1 refrigerated pie crust (un-baked)

Egg Base:

- 6 eggs
- 1/3 cup heavy cream
- 1/4 tsp salt
- 1/4 tsp chicken bouillon powder (optional)
- 1/4 tsp black pepper

Toppings:

- 1/4 cup breakfast sausage (uncooked)
- 1/4 cup ham (chopped)
- 1 1/2 cups cheddar cheese

Instructions

1. Preheat the oven to 350°F. Unroll 1 pie crust onto a pie dish and crimp the edges. Set aside.
2. Meanwhile, whisk together the eggs, cream, chicken bouillon powder, salt, and pepper. Pour into the prepared crust.
3. Sprinkle the sausage and ham over the eggs. Top with cheese (about 1 1/2" thick) and bake for 30-40 minutes or until the center puffs out like a dome.
4. Cool slightly. Cut into 8 slices and serve.

Prep Time: 10 Minutes

Cook Time: 5 Minutes

Servings: 12

Ingredients

- 12-inch cast-iron skillet
- Spatula
- 6 slices bacon
- 6 eggs
- 1/4 cup milk
- 6 wheat tortillas (large 10-inch tortillas)
- 2 cups Monterey Jack Colby Cheese (grated)

Instructions

1. In a cast-iron skillet over medium heat, fry the bacon slices until crisp.
2. Meanwhile, whisk the eggs, milk, and salt, and pepper to taste.
3. how to make breakfast quesadillas

4. When bacon is done remove it from the pan and pour in the beaten eggs. Cook until scrambled and cooked thoroughly.

5. how to assemble a breakfast quesadilla

6. Remove the eggs with a slotted spoon and wipe clean the pan. Keep pre-heated over medium heat while you assemble the quesadillas.

7. Arrange three flour tortillas over the countertop and evenly divide with cheese, scrambled eggs, and bacon pieces. Top with the other three tortillas and toast each quesadilla on both sides in the preheated pan for 1-2 minutes.

8. how to cut a quesadilla into wedges

9. Slice each quesadilla into fours and serve with sour cream, Pico De Gallo, or salsa.

Prep Time: 5 Minutes

Cook Time: 15 Minutes

Servings: 12

Ingredients

French Toast:

- 1 cup milk
- 1/4 cup all-purpose flour
- 3 eggs
- 1 tsp ground cinnamon
- 1 TBSP sugar
- 1/8 tsp salt
- 1 French Bread Baguette thickly sliced

Instructions

1. Pre-heat skillet over med-low heat with 1/3 cup of oil. Place flour and spices into a bowl and slowly whisk in the milk.
2. Add the eggs and mix well.

3. Dip each slice of bread in the mixture for about 2-3 seconds on each side. Fry in skillet for 3-4 minutes on each side.

4. Fry in skillet for 3-4 minutes on each side.

Prep Time: 5 Minutes

Cook Time: 25 Minutes

Servings: 23

Ingredients

- 12-inch non-stick skillet

For Sourdough English Muffins:

- 1 1/2 cups sourdough starter (active)
- 3 cups milk
- 4 Tbsp honey
- 6 cups white whole wheat flour
- 1 Tbsp salt
- 4 tsp baking soda

Instructions

1. How to make Sourdough English Muffins:
2. In a large bowl mix the starter, milk, honey, and flour together. Cover and leave overnight at room

temperature. (It's best to do this at night or rest for a minimum of 10 hours.)

3. In the morning, knead in the salt and baking soda until smooth.

4. Pre-heat a skillet over med-low heat (300°F.)

5. how to make english muffins with whole wheat flour and dredge in cornmeal

6. To make English muffins: scoop 1/3 cup of dough and form into a ball. Lightly dredge the top and bottom with fine cornmeal and transfer into a tray dusted with cornmeal. Repeat until all muffins are done.

7. how to cook english muffins

8. Fry English Muffins covered, (no oil needed) for 3-5 minutes on each side or until done and no longer doughy in the inside.

9. Split open and serve toasted with butter and jam!

Prep Time: 5 Minutes

Cook Time: 25 Minutes

Servings: 6

Ingredients

- 10 or 12-inch cast-iron pan
- 1 1/2 lbs large raw shrimp (thawed and patted dry)
- 1 Tbsp unsalted butter
- 1 Tbsp olive oil
- 3 cups mozzarella cheese
- 6 large flour tortillas

Seasoning:

- 5 cloves garlic (crushed)
- 1/4 tsp garlic salt
- 1/4 tsp seasoning salt
- 1/2 tsp creole seasoning
- 1/2 tsp old bay seasoning

Instructions

1. Preheat a cast-iron skillet with butter and olive oil over medium heat.
2. Season the shrimp evenly on both sides. Fry on each side until shrimp turns pink (2 minutes.)
3. Remove the shrimp and place the skillet back on the stove. Add an additional 2 tbsp of grease and reduce the temperature to low heat.
4. To Assemble Quesadillas: coarsely chop the cooked shrimp. Place 1/2 cup of mozzarella and 1/2 cup the shrimp evenly over a large tortilla. Fold in half and toast on each side until the cheese melts.

Prep Time: 2hrs 5 Minutes

Cook Time: 1hrs 25 Minutes

Servings: 8

Ingredients

- 1 (16-ounce) loaf brioche bread, cubed
- 1 (8-ounce) package cream cheese, cubed
- 1 pound strawberries, diced and divided
- 12 large eggs, beaten
- 2 cups whole milk
- 1/3 cup maple syrup
- 1 teaspoon vanilla extract
- 1/2 teaspoon kosher salt
- 1 tablespoon confectioners' sugar

Instructions

1. Lightly coat a 9×13 baking dish with nonstick spray. Place a layer of bread cubes evenly into the baking dish. Top with cream cheese and half the strawberries

in an even layer. Top with remaining bread cubes to completely cover the filling.

2. In a large glass measuring cup or another bowl, whisk together eggs, milk, maple syrup, vanilla and salt. Pour mixture evenly over the bread cubes. Cover and place in the refrigerator for at least 2 hours or overnight.

3. Preheat oven to 350 degrees F. Remove baking dish from the refrigerator; let stand 30 minutes.

4. Place into oven and bake, covered, for 30 minutes. Uncover; continue to bake for an additional 25-30 minutes, or until golden brown and center is firm.

5. Serve immediately, sprinkled with remaining strawberries and confectioners' sugar, if desired.

Prep Time: 25 Minutes

Cook Time: 1hrs 15 Minutes

Servings: 8

Ingredients

- 1 (16-ounce) loaf sourdough bread, cut into 1-inch cubes
- 1 tablespoon olive oil
- 1 pound breakfast sausage
- 4 tablespoons unsalted butter
- 3 cloves garlic, minced
- 1 sweet onion, diced
- 2 celery ribs, diced
- 2 tablespoons chopped fresh parsley leaves
- 2 tablespoons chopped fresh sage leaves
- 1 ½ tablespoons chopped fresh thyme leaves
- 2 teaspoons chopped fresh rosemary
- salt and freshly ground black pepper, to taste
- 2 ½ cups chicken stock

Instructions

1. Preheat oven to 400 degrees F. Lightly oil a 9 x 13 baking dish or coat with nonstick spray.

2. Spread bread cubes in a single layer on a baking sheet. Place into oven and bake until crisp and golden, about 10-13 minutes; set aside.

3. Heat olive oil in a large cast iron skillet over medium heat. Add sausage and cook until browned, about 5-8 minutes, making sure to crumble the sausage as it cooks. Transfer sausage to a paper towel-lined plate.

4. Melt butter in the skillet. Add garlic, onion and celery, and cook, stirring occasionally, until tender, about 4-5 minutes. Stir in parsley, sage, thyme and rosemary until fragrant, about 1 minute.

5. Remove from heat. Stir in bread and sausage; season with salt and pepper, to taste. Stir in chicken stock until absorbed and well combined. Let stand 5 minutes, stirring occasionally, until liquid is absorbed.*

6. Spread bread mixture into the prepared baking dish. Place into oven and bake until top is browned, about 30-35 minutes.

7. Serve immediately.

Prep Time: 2hrs 25 Minutes

Cook Time: 1hrs 10 Minutes

Servings: 8

Ingredients

- 1 1/4 pounds fresh croissants (about 12 medium), cut in half
- 1 (8-ounce) package cream cheese, cubed
- 2 1/2 cups fresh raspberries
- 12 large eggs, beaten
- 2 cups whole milk
- 1/4 cup honey
- 1 teaspoon vanilla extract
- 1/2 teaspoon kosher salt
- 1 tablespoon confectioners' sugar

Instructions

1. Lightly coat a 9×13 baking dish with nonstick spray. Place half of croissants evenly into the baking dish. Top with half of cream cheese and 3/4 cup raspberries

in an even layer. Top with remaining croissants, cream cheese and 3/4 cup raspberries.

2. In a large glass measuring cup or another bowl, whisk together eggs, milk, honey, vanilla and salt. Pour mixture evenly over the croissants. Cover and place in the refrigerator for at least 2 hours or overnight.

3. Preheat oven to 350 degrees F. Remove baking dish from the refrigerator; let stand 30 minutes.

4. Place into oven and bake, covered, for 30 minutes. Uncover; continue to bake for an additional 30-35 minutes, or until golden brown and center is firm.

5. Serve immediately, sprinkled with remaining raspberries and confectioners' sugar, if desired.

Prep Time: 15 Minutes

Cook Time: 30 Minutes

Servings: 10

Ingredients

- 4-quart pot
- wooden spoon
- 1 onion diced
- 10 oz mild sausage (2 1/2 sausage links casings removed)
- 6 slices pre-cooked bacon (chopped)
- 2 garlic cloves (crushed)
- 12 cups water
- 1 tbsp salt
- 1 tsp chicken bouillon powder
- 6 potatoes, chopped (skins on and washed)
- 1 1/4 cup heavy cream
- 1 bunch kale (leaves stripped and chopped)
- 1/2 tsp cayenne pepper

Instructions

1. potatoes, bacon, heavy cream, cayenne pepper, chicken bouillon, salt, water, fresh kale, onion, Italian pork sausage, and garlic

2. In a large pot; saute the onion, sausage, bacon, and garlic for 7 minutes.

3. how to make Zuppa Toscana in one-pot. Step 1: fry the onion, Italian sausage, bacon, and garlic first.

4. Add the water, salt, and chicken bouillon powder: bring to a boil. Add the potatoes and simmer for 25 minutes.

5. How to make Zuppa Toscana in one-pot. Step 2: Add the water, salt, chicken bouillon, and potatoes. Simmer for 25 minutes.

6. Stir in the cream, kale, and cayenne pepper. Bring to a boil and turn soup off.

7. How to make Zuppa Toscana in one-pot. Step 3: Stir in the cream, kale, and cayenne pepper; bring to a boil and remove from heat.

8. Garnish soup with freshly grated parmesan cheese before serving!

Prep Time: 5 Minutes

Cook Time: 10 Minutes

Servings: 10

Ingredients

- 5-quart pot
- Broccoli Cheese Soup:
- 2 Tbsp butter
- 3 Tbsp onions (chopped)
- 5 Tbsp flour
- 1 lb cubed processed cheese (Velveeta)
- 5 1/2 cups half and half
- 1/2 tsp salt
- 1/2 tsp chicken bullion
- 1 tsp ground mustard
- 1/2 tsp black pepper
- 1/4 tsp dried onion
- 10 oz frozen broccoli
- French's French Fried Onions (optional garnish)

Instructions

1. Fry the onion in butter in a medium-sized pot for 1 minute over high. Whisk in the flour then add 1 1/2 cups of half and half and scrape off any debris. Whisk in the cheese and stir until mostly melted.
2. Add the remaining ingredients except for the french fried onion chips and bring to boil stirring often. Simmer until broccoli is heated thoroughly.
3. Ladle into soup bowls and sprinkle with french fried onions. Serve.

Prep Time: 50 Minutes

Cook Time: 2hrs 10 Minutes

Servings: 25

Ingredients

- 22x12" pan
- 8-quart pot
- large mixing bowl

Cabbage Rolls:

- 5 lbs ground pork
- 2 heads cabbage (or 1 XL Cabbage)
- 11/2 cups uncooked rice
- 24 oz pasta sauce
- 1 onion
- 2 carrots
- 4 tbsp olive oil
- 2 tbsp salt
- 11/2 tsp ground black pepper
- 3 cups water (divided)
- 10 bay leaves

Instructions

How To Make Cabbage Rolls:

1. Combine the rice and 1 1/2 cups of water. Bring to a boil then remove from heat and allow to sit covered for 5 minutes.
2. Meanwhile, grate the carrots and onion; fry in olive oil until browned (8 min.)
3. Remove the core of the cabbage. Boil the cabbage for 5 minutes covered. Then remove the outer leaves that have been loosened and repeat in 3-minute increments until done.
4. In a large bowl combine the rice, carrot mixture, ground pork, salt, and pepper. Mix and set aside.
5. Trim the stems and cut the bigger cabbage leaves in half. Place a heaping tablespoon of filling into each leaf and roll up tucking in the sides. Place seam down into a baking dish.
6. Spread the bay leaves over the cabbage rolls. Dilute the pasta sauce with the remaining 1 1/2 cups water and pour over the rolls.
7. Cover and bake at 370°F for 2 hours.

Prep Time: 20 Minutes

Cook Time: 20 Minutes

Servings: 4

Ingredients

- 2 tablespoons olive oil, divided
- 3 cloves garlic, minced
- 1 onion, diced
- 3 carrots, peeled and diced
- 2 stalks celery, diced
- ½ teaspoon dried thyme
- 5 cups chicken stock
- 2 bay leaves
- 2 cups baby spinach
- ¼ cup freshly grated Parmesan cheese
- 2 tablespoons chopped fresh parsley leaves

For The Meatballs:

- 1 pound ground turkey
- ⅓ cup Panko
- ¼ cup freshly grated Parmesan cheese

- ½ teaspoon dried oregano
- ½ teaspoon dried basil
- ½ teaspoon dried parsley
- ¼ teaspoon garlic powder
- ¼ teaspoon crushed red pepper flakes
- salt and freshly ground black pepper, to taste

Instructions

1. In a large bowl, combine ground turkey, Panko, Parmesan, oregano, basil, parsley, garlic powder and red pepper flakes; season with salt and pepper, to taste. Using a wooden spoon or clean hands, stir until well combined. Roll the mixture into 1 1/4-to-1 1/2-inch meatballs, forming about 18-20 meatballs.

2. Heat 1 tablespoon olive oil in a large stockpot or Dutch oven over medium heat. Add meatballs, in batches, and cook until all sides are browned, about 2-3 minutes. Transfer to a paper towel-lined plate; set aside.

3. Add remaining 1 tablespoon olive oil to the skillet. Add garlic, onion, carrots and celery. Cook, stirring occasionally, until tender, about 3-4 minutes. Stir in thyme until fragrant, about 1 minute.

4. Whisk in chicken stock, bay leaves and 1 cup water; bring to a boil. Stir in meatballs; reduce heat and simmer until meatballs are cooked through, about 10-12 minutes. Stir in spinach until wilted, about 2 minutes.

5. Serve immediately, sprinkled with Parmesan and garnished with parsley, if desired.

Prep Time: 15 Minutes

Cook Time: 10 Minutes

Servings: 4

Ingredients

- ½ cup vegetable oil
- 1 pound boneless, skinless chicken breasts, cut into 1-inch chunks
- Kosher salt and freshly ground black pepper, to taste
- 1 cup Panko
- ¼ cup freshly grated Parmesan
- 1 teaspoon garlic powder
- ½ teaspoon smoked paprika
- ½ cup all-purpose flour
- 2 large eggs, beaten
- 2 tablespoons chopped fresh parsley leaves

Instructions

1. Heat vegetable oil in a large skillet over medium high heat.

2. Season chicken with salt and pepper, to taste.

3. In a large bowl, combine Panko, Parmesan, garlic powder and smoked paprika; season with salt and pepper, to taste. Set aside.

4. Working in batches, dredge chicken in flour, dip into eggs, then dredge in Panko mixture, pressing to coat.

5. Add chicken to the skillet, 5 or 6 at a time, and cook until evenly golden and crispy, about 3-4 minutes. Transfer to a paper towel-lined plate.

6. Serve immediately, garnished with Parmesan and parsley, if desired.

16. Cpk's Kung Pao Spaghetti

Prep Time: 15 Minutes

Cook Time: 10 Minutes

Servings: 4

Ingredients

- 1 pound spaghetti
- 2 tablespoons vegetable oil
- 3 boneless, skinless thin-sliced chicken breasts
- Kosher salt and freshly ground black pepper, to taste
- 4 cloves garlic, minced
- ½ cup dry roasted peanuts
- 2 green onions, thinly sliced

For The Sauce:

- ½ cup reduced sodium soy sauce
- ½ cup chicken broth
- ½ cup dry sherry
- 2 tablespoons red chili paste with garlic, or more, to taste
- ¼ cup sugar
- 2 tablespoons red wine vinegar

- 2 tablespoons cornstarch
- 1 tablespoon sesame oil

Instructions

1. In a small bowl, whisk together soy sauce, chicken broth, dry sherry, red chili paste, sugar, red wine vinegar, cornstarch and sesame oil; set aside.
2. In a large pot of boiling salted water, cook pasta according to package instructions; drain well.
3. Heat vegetable oil in a large skillet over medium high heat. Season chicken breasts with salt and pepper, to taste. Add to skillet and cook, flipping once, until cooked through, about 3-4 minutes per side. Let cool before dicing into bite-size pieces; set aside.
4. Add garlic to the skillet and cook, stirring constantly, until fragrant, about 1 minute. Stir in soy sauce mixture and bring to a boil; reduce heat and simmer until thickened, about 1-2 minutes. Stir in pasta, chicken, peanuts and green onions.
5. Serve immediately.

Prep Time: 10 Minutes

Cook Time: 25 Minutes

Servings: 6

Ingredients

- 2 teaspoons olive oil
- ¼ cup Panko
- 8 ounces Cream Cheese, at room temperature
- 2 ½ cups fresh broccoli florets
- ¾ cup shredded cheddar cheese, divided
- ½ cup sour cream
- ¼ cup grated Parmesan
- ¼ cup milk
- 1 tablespoon Emeril's Essence Creole Seasoning
- ½ teaspoon garlic powder
- ½ teaspoon onion powder
- salt and freshly ground black pepper, to taste

Instructions

1. Preheat oven to 375 degrees F. Lightly oil a 9-inch baking dish or coat with nonstick spray.

2. Heat olive oil in a large skillet over medium high heat. Add Panko and cook, stirring, until browned and toasted, about 3 minutes; set aside.

3. In a large bowl, combine cream cheese, broccoli, 1/2 cup cheddar cheese, sour cream, Parmesan, milk, Emeril's Essence, garlic powder and onion powder; season with salt and pepper, to taste.

4. Spread broccoli mixture into the prepared baking dish; sprinkle with remaining 1/4 cup cheddar cheese. Place into oven and bake until bubbly, about 20-25 minutes.

5. Serve immediately, sprinkled with Panko, if desired.

Prep Time: 10 Minutes

Cook Time: 25 Minutes

Servings: 4

Ingredients

- 16 ounces extra wide egg noodles
- 1 ¼ cups enchilada sauce
- 1 cup canned corn kernels, drained
- 1 cup canned black beans, drained and rinsed
- 1 cup shredded cheddar cheese, divided
- 1 cup shredded Monterey Jack cheese, divided
- ¼ cup Greek yogurt
- 1 4-ounce can diced green chiles
- 1 tablespoon olive oil
- 1 pound ground beef
- 4 ounces cream cheese
- ½ teaspoon chili powder, or more to taste
- ¼ teaspoon cumin
- salt and freshly ground black pepper, to taste
- 1 avocado, halved, seeded, peeled and diced
- 2 tablespoons chopped fresh cilantro leaves

Instructions

1. Preheat oven to 350 degrees F. Lightly oil a 9×13 baking dish or coat with nonstick spray.
2. In a large pot of boiling salted water, cook pasta according to package instructions; drain well.
3. In a large bowl, combine enchilada sauce, corn, beans, 1/2 cup cheddar cheese, 1/2 cup Monterey Jack cheese, Greek yogurt and green chiles; set aside.
4. Heat olive oil in a saucepan over medium high heat. Add ground beef and cook until browned, about 3-5 minutes, making sure to crumble the beef as it cooks; drain excess fat.
5. Stir in cream cheese, chili powder and cumin until cream cheese has melted. Stir in pasta and enchilada mixture until well combined; season with salt and pepper, to taste.
6. Add pasta to prepared baking dish and top with avocado and remaining cheeses. Place into oven and bake until cheeses have melted, about 5-10 minutes.
7. Serve immediately, garnished with cilantro.

Prep Time: 10 Minutes

Cook Time: 5 Minutes

Servings: 4

Ingredients

- 1 tablespoon olive oil
- 2 boneless, skinless thin-sliced chicken breasts
- salt and freshly ground black pepper, to taste
- 6 cups chopped romaine lettuce
- 1 Roma tomato, diced
- ¾ cup canned corn kernels, drained
- ¾ cup canned black beans, drained and rinsed
- ¼ cup diced red onion
- ¼ cup shredded Monterey Jack cheese
- ½ cup shredded cheddar cheese
- ¼ cup Ranch dressing
- ¼ cup BBQ sauce
- ¼ cup tortilla strips

Instructions

1. Heat olive oil in a medium skillet over medium high heat.
2. Season chicken breasts with salt and pepper, to taste. Add to skillet and cook, flipping once, until cooked through, about 3-4 minutes per side. Let cool before dicing into bite-size pieces.
3. To assemble the salad, place romaine lettuce in a large bowl; top with chicken, tomato, corn, beans, onion and cheeses. Pour Ranch dressing and BBQ sauce on top of the salad and gently toss to combine.
4. Serve immediately, topped with tortilla strips.

Prep Time: 10 Minutes

Cook Time: 45 Minutes

Servings: 4

Ingredients

- 2 tablespoons unsalted butter
- 1 large leek, thinly sliced
- 1 large red bell pepper, diced
- 2 cups milk
- 3 tablespoons all-purpose flour
- 3 cups vegetable broth
- 2 cups roasted corn kernels
- 2 pounds red potatoes, cubed
- 1 ½ teaspoons Emeril's Essence Creole Seasoning
- ¾ teaspoon thyme
- ¾ teaspoon salt
- Chopped fresh chives, for garnish

For Emeril's Essence Creole Seasoning:

- 2 ½ tablespoons paprika
- 2 tablespoons garlic powder

- 2 tablespoons salt
- 1 tablespoon onion powder
- 1 tablespoon cayenne pepper
- 1 tablespoon oregano
- 1 tablespoon thyme
- 1 tablespoon black pepper

Instructions

1. To make Emeril's Essence, combine paprika, garlic powder, salt, onion powder, cayenne pepper, oregano, thyme and pepper; set aside.
2. Melt butter in a large stockpot or Dutch oven over medium heat. Add leeks and bell pepper, and cook, stirring occasionally, until tender, about 5 minutes. Gradually whisk in milk and flour, and cook, whisking constantly, until incorporated, about 1-2 minutes. Stir in vegetable broth, corn kernels, potatoes, 1 1/2 teaspoons Emeril's Essence, thyme and salt.
3. Bring to a boil; reduce heat and simmer until potatoes are tender, about 20-30 minutes.
4. Serve immediately, garnished with chives.

21. Baked Tomato Bruschetta

Prep Time: 10 Minutes

Cook Time: 15 Minutes

Servings: 4

Ingredients

- 1 baguette, thinly sliced
- 3 tablespoons olive oil, divided
- 4 slices Sargento Mozzarella Cheese
- 2 cups cherry tomatoes, halved
- 1 teaspoon balsamic vinegar
- 1 clove garlic, pressed
- Pinch of kosher salt
- Pinch of freshly ground black pepper
- ¼ cup basil leaves, chiffonade

Instructions

1. Preheat oven to 350 degrees F. Line a baking sheet with parchment paper.

2. Place baguette slices onto prepared baking sheet. Drizzle with 2 tablespoons olive oil. Place into oven and bake for 8-10 minutes, or until golden brown.

3. Top each baguette slice with mozzarella cheese. Place into oven and bake for 4-6 minutes, or until cheese has melted.

4. In a large bowl, combine tomatoes, remaining 1 tablespoon olive oil, balsamic vinegar, garlic, salt and pepper, to taste.

5. Top each baguette slice with tomato mixture, garnished with basil.

6. Serve immediately.

22. Zucchini Parmesan Foil Packets

Prep Time: 10 Minutes

Cook Time: 15 Minutes

Servings: 4

Ingredients

- ¼ cup unsalted butter, melted
- ¼ cup freshly grated Parmesan
- 1 teaspoon dried basil
- 1 teaspoon dried oregano
- salt and freshly ground black pepper, to taste
- 4 zucchini, cut into 1/4-inch thick rounds
- ¼ teaspoon crushed red pepper flakes
- 2 tablespoons chopped fresh parsley leaves

Instructions

1. PREHEAT a gas or charcoal grill over high heat.
2. WHISK together butter, Parmesan, basil and oregano; season with salt and pepper, to taste.
3. CENTER zucchini on a sheet of Reynolds Wrap® Heavy Duty Foil. Spoon butter mixture over zucchini.

Bring up foil sides. Double fold top and ends to seal packet, leaving room for heat circulation inside.

4. PLACE foil packets on the grill and cook until just cooked through, about 15-20 minutes.

5. SERVE immediately, garnished with red pepper flakes and parsley, if desired.

Prep Time: 10 Minutes

Cook Time: 4hrs 15 Minutes

Servings: 8

Ingredients

- ¼ cup brown sugar, packed
- 3 cloves garlic, minced
- ½ teaspoon dried rosemary
- Kosher salt and freshly ground black pepper, to taste
- 1 3-pound boneless pork loin, excess fat trimmed
- 2 tablespoons vegetable oil
- 6 slices bacon
- 1 sprig rosemary

For The Glaze:

- ¼ cup fig jam
- 2 tablespoons Dijon mustard
- 1 tablespoon whole grain mustard
- Zest of 1 orange

Instructions

1. In a small bowl, combine fig jam, mustards and orange zest; set aside.

2. In a small bowl, combine brown sugar, garlic, rosemary, salt and pepper. Season pork loin with brown sugar mixture, rubbing in thoroughly on all sides.

3. Heat vegetable oil in a large skillet over medium high heat. Add pork loin, and sear both sides until golden brown, about 2-3 minutes per side.

4. Starting on 1 side, lay a slice of bacon, crosswise, on top of the pork, laying another slice to slightly overlap the first. Continue with remaining slices until fully covered.

5. Place pork loin into a 6-qt slow cooker; top with fig jam mixture. Cover and cook on low heat for 3-4 hours, or until completely cooked through, reaching an internal temperature of 140 degrees F.

6. Serve immediately, garnished with rosemary, if desired.

Prep Time: 10 Minutes

Cook Time: 30 Minutes

Servings: 4

Ingredients

- 3 tablespoons olive oil
- 1 tablespoon Dijon mustard
- 1 tablespoon whole grain mustard
- ½ teaspoon dried thyme
- ¼ teaspoon dried rosemary
- Zest of 1 lemon
- salt and freshly ground black pepper, to taste
- 16 ounces baby red potatoes, halved
- Kosher salt and freshly ground black pepper, to taste
- 4 boneless, skinless chicken breasts
- 1 lemon, thinly sliced
- 2 tablespoons chopped fresh parsley leaves

Instructions

1. Preheat oven to 375 degrees F.

2. In a small bowl, combine 2 tablespoons olive oil, mustards, thyme, rosemary and lemon zest; season with salt and pepper, to taste. Set aside.

3. Cut four sheets of foil, about 12-inches long. Divide potatoes into 4 equal portions and add to the center of each foil in a single layer.

4. Fold up all 4 sides of each foil packet. Drizzle with remaining 1 tablespoon olive oil and season with salt and pepper, to taste; gently toss to combine.

5. Top each packet with the chicken. Using your fingers or a brush, work the mustard mixture onto both sides of the chicken. Top with lemon slices.

6. Fold the sides of the foil over the chicken, covering completely and sealing the packets closed. Place foil packets in a single layer on a baking sheet. Place into oven and bake until the chicken is cooked through and the potatoes are tender, about 25-30 minutes.

7. OPTIONAL: Preheat oven to broil. Open the packets and broil for 2-3 minutes, or until caramelized and slightly charred.

8. Served immediately, garnished with parsley, if desired.

Prep Time: 30 Minutes

Cook Time: 30 Minutes

Servings: 6

Ingredients

- 2 tablespoons olive oil, divded
- 1 onion, thinly sliced
- 1 red bell pepper, thinly sliced
- 1 orange bell pepper, thinly sliced
- 1 green bell pepper, thinly sliced
- 8 cups chopped romaine lettuce
- 1 avocado, halved, seeded, peeled and thinly sliced

For The Cilantro Lime Dressing

- 1 cup loosely packed cilantro, stems removed
- ½ cup sour cream
- 2 tablespoons mayonnaise
- 2 cloves garlic
- Juice of 1 lime
- Pinch of salt
- ¼ cup olive oil

- 2 tablespoons apple cider vinegar

For The Steak:

- ¼ cup olive oil
- 2 cloves garlic, minced
- Juice of 1 lime
- 1 teaspoon ground cumin
- 1 teaspoon chili powder
- 1 teaspoon dried oregano
- ½ teaspoon onion powder
- salt and freshly ground black pepper
- 2 pounds flank steak

Instructions

1. To make the cilantro lime dressing, combine cilantro, sour cream, mayonnaise, garlic, lime juice and salt in the bowl of a food processor. With the motor running, add olive oil and vinegar in a slow stream until emulsified; set aside.

2. To make the steak, whisk together olive oil, garlic, lime juice, cumin, chili powder, oregano and onion powder in a small bowl; season with salt and pepper, to taste.

3. In a gallon size Ziploc bag or large bowl, combine steak and marinade; marinate for at least 30 minutes, turning the bag occasionally. Drain the steak from the marinade, discarding the marinade.

4. Heat 1 tablespoon olive oil in a grill pan over medium high heat. Working in batches, cook steak, flipping once, to preferred temperature, about 3-4 minutes per side for medium rare. Remove from heat and let rest for 10 minutes before thinly slicing against the grain.

5. Add onion to the skillet, and cook, stirring often, until onions have become translucent and slightly caramelized, about 7-8 minutes; set aside.

6. Heat remaining 1 tablespoon olive oil in the skillet. Add bell peppers, and cook, stirring often, until soft and slightly caramelized, about 8-10 minutes; set aside.

7. To assemble the salad, place romaine lettuce in a large bowl; top with arranged rows of onion, peppers, steak and avocado.

8. Serve immediately with cilantro lime dressing.

Prep Time: 1hrs 10 Minutes

Cook Time: 1hrs 15 Minutes

Servings: 4

Ingredients

- 1 pound tilapia fillets, cut in half lengthwise
- Kosher salt and freshly ground black pepper, to taste
- 2 limes, juiced
- 4 cloves garlic, minced
- 2 tablespoons unsalted butter
- 8 taco shells
- 1 cup shredded red cabbage
- 2 avocados, halved, seeded, peeled and diced
- 2 Roma tomatoes, diced
- 2 tablespoons fresh chopped cilantro leaves

For The Chipotle Mayo

- ¼ cup mayonnaise
- ¼ cup Greek yogurt
- 1 tablespoon chipotle paste
- 1 tablespoon freshly squeezed lime juice

- 2 cloves garlic, pressed

Instructions

1. To make the chipotle mayo, whisk together mayonnaise, Greek yogurt, chipotle paste, lime juice and garlic; set aside.
2. Season tilapia with salt and pepper, to taste.
3. In a shallow bowl, marinate tilapia with lime juice and garlic for at least 1 hour.
4. Melt butter in a large skillet over medium high heat. Add tilapia and cook, flipping once, until golden brown, about 2-3 minutes per side.
5. To serve, spoon tilapia into the center of each taco shell. Top with cabbage, avocados, tomatoes and cilantro, drizzled with chipotle mayo.

Prep Time: 10 Minutes

Cook Time: 35 Minutes

Servings: 4

Ingredients

- 1 pound spaghetti
- 2 boneless, skinless chicken breasts, cut crosswise in half
- ¾ cup Italian style breadcrumbs
- ¼ cup grated Parmesan cheese
- 2 tablespoons unsalted butter, melted
- ¾ cup shredded mozzarella cheese
- 1 cup marinara sauce, homemade or storebought

Instructions

1. Preheat oven to 450 degrees F. Line a baking sheet with parchment paper or a silicone baking mat; set aside.
2. In a large pot of boiling salted water, cook pasta according to package instructions; drain well.

3. In a small bowl, combine breadcrumbs and Parmesan. Working one at a time, brush butter on each chicken breast and dredge in breadcrumb mixture, pressing to coat.

4. Place onto prepared baking sheet and bake for 20 minutes. Gently flip and bake until the crust is golden and the chicken is completely cooked through, about 5 minutes more.

5. Remove from oven; spoon 1 tablespoon marinara on each chicken breast and sprinkle with 1-2 tablespoons mozzarella. Place into oven and bake until cheese has melted, about 5 minutes.

6. Serve immediately with spaghetti and additional marinara, if desired.

Prep Time: 5 Minutes

Cook Time: 15 Minutes

Servings: 4

Ingredients

- ¼ cup brown sugar, packed
- ¼ cup reduced sodium soy sauce
- 2 teaspoons sesame oil
- ½ teaspoon crushed red-pepper flakes, or more to taste
- ¼ teaspoon ground ginger
- 1 tablespoon vegetable oil
- 3 cloves garlic, minced
- 1 pound ground beef
- 2 green onions, thinly sliced
- ¼ teaspoon sesame seeds

Instructions

1. In a small bowl, whisk together brown sugar, soy sauce, sesame oil, red pepper flakes and ginger.

2. Heat vegetable oil in a large skillet over medium high heat. Add garlic and cook, stirring constantly, until fragrant, about 1 minute. Add ground beef and cook until browned, about 3-5 minutes, making sure to crumble the beef as it cooks; drain excess fat.

3. Stir in soy sauce mixture and green onions until well combined, allowing to simmer until heated through, about 2 minutes.

4. Serve immediately, garnished with green onion and sesame seeds, if desired.

Prep Time: 15 Minutes

Cook Time: 15 Minutes

Servings: 4

Ingredients

- 8 ounces elbows pasta
- 1 California Avocado, halved, seeded, peeled and diced
- 1 mango, peeled and diced
- 1 carrot, peeled and grated
- ¼ cup shredded red cabbage
- 1 green onion, thinly sliced
- 2 tablespoons pine nuts
- salt and freshly ground black pepper, to taste

For The Dressing:

- 2 tablespoons soy sauce
- 2 teaspoons sesame oil
- 1 ½ teaspoons sugar, or more to taste
- ½ teaspoon sesame seeds

Instructions

1. To make the dressing, whisk together soy sauce, sesame oil, sugar and sesame seeds; set aside.
2. In a large pot of boiling salted water, cook pasta according to package instructions; drain well.
3. In a large bowl, combine pasta, avocado, mango, carrot, cabbage, green onion, pine nut, soy sauce dressing, salt and pepper to taste.
4. Serve immediately.

Prep Time: 20 Minutes

Cook Time: 15 Minutes

Servings: 60

Ingredients

Spread:

- 10 oz cream cheese softened
- 3 Tbsp banana peppers chopped
- 1 Tbsp Italian dressing mix
- 1/4 cup onion diced
- 1/3 cup red bell pepper diced
- 1/2 cup mozzarella cheese grated

Pinwheels:

- 10 tortillas burrito size
- 10 slices ham
- 5 oz pepperoni
- 10 slices provolone cheese

Instructions

1. In a small bowl beat cream cheese, banana peppers, Italian dressing mix, onion, red bell pepper and mozzarella cheese until well combined.
2. Spread cream cheese mixture over a burrito sized tortilla.
3. Layer ham, pepperoni and cheese over the spread and roll-up.
4. Cut each tortilla into 6 equal pieces. Serve immediately or keep refrigerated.

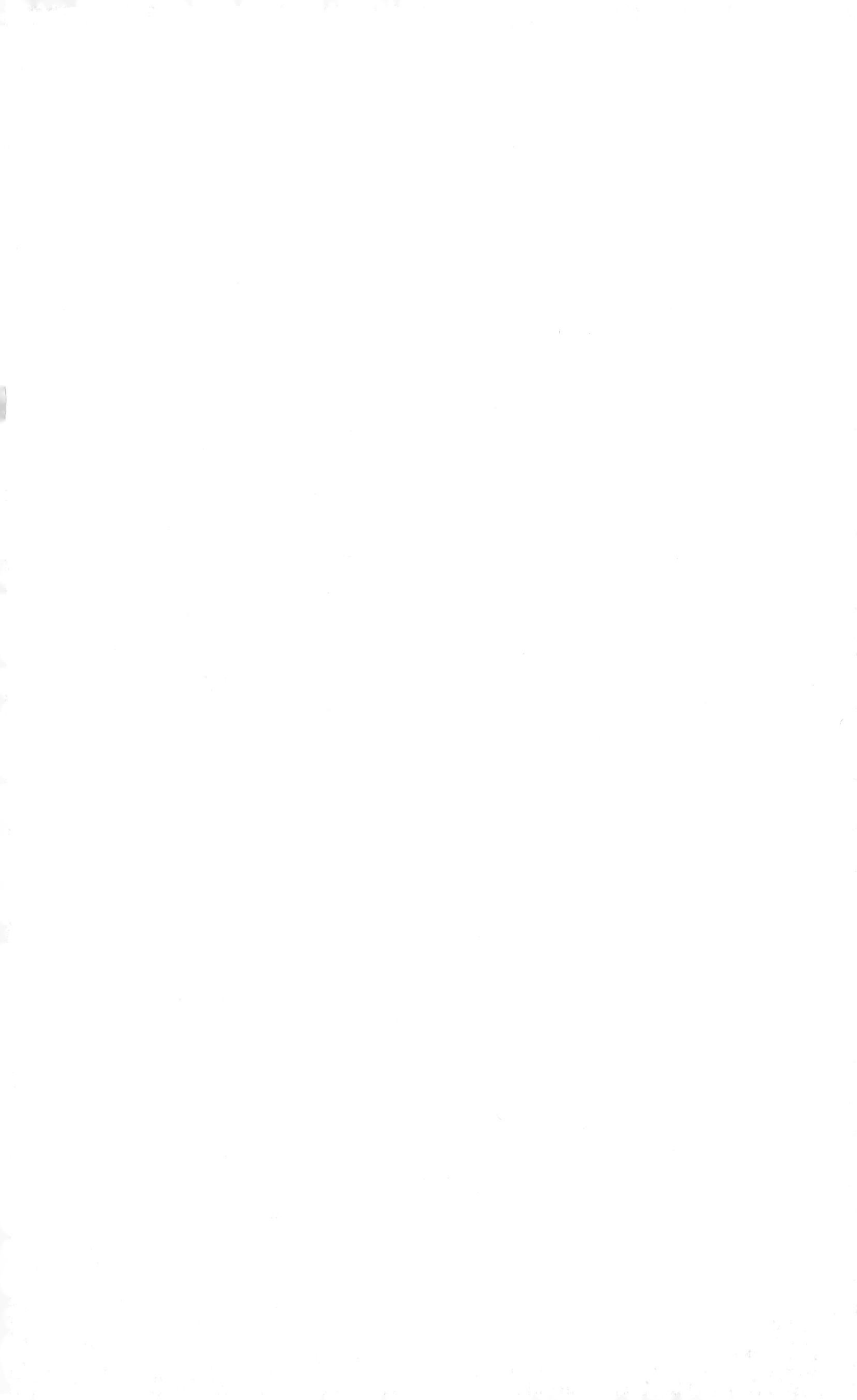